THE HEALTHY WAY:

A GUIDE TO LONG-TERM WEIGHT MANAGEMENT

BY

Dr. CAMELLIA FENNIMORE

CONTENTS

INTRODUCTION

This book is not a "diet" or a "program" that will lead to healthy weight loss, but rather a lifestyle change that includes healthy eating patterns, frequent physical activity, and effective stress management. Medications taken for the treatment of other ailments may also make it more difficult to shed excess pounds.

It's only normal to want to see results as quickly as possible when you're trying to get rid of excess weight. People who lose weight slowly and consistently (approximately one to two pounds per week) have a greater chance of successfully maintaining their weight loss.

After you have reached a healthy weight for your height, you can rely on a nutritious diet and regular exercise to assist you in maintaining your health over the long term.

It's not easy to lose weight, and it takes dedication to do it. However, if you are ready to get started, we have a step-by-step guide that will assist you in getting started on the path to a healthier lifestyle and reduced body weight. Before beginning the guide, it is essential to have a self-compassionate attitude toward the adjustments, as well as an understanding of your preparation and motivation. You may improve your chances of achieving your goals by cultivating a setting that is encouraging, both in terms of the physical surroundings and the relationships you maintain.

Even a moderate amount of weight loss can result in significant improvements.
There is a good chance that you may experience improvements in your blood pressure, blood cholesterol levels, and blood sugar levels after losing as little as five percent to ten percent of your total body weight.

If you weigh 200 pounds, for instance, a 5% weight loss would be 10 pounds, reducing your weight down to 190 pounds from its previous level of 200 pounds. Despite the fact that this weight may still place a person in the category of "overweight" or "obesity," even a slight reduction in weight might help reduce the chance of developing chronic diseases that are linked to obesity.

Therefore, even though the overall objective seems to be quite ambitious, you should look at it more as a process than as an endpoint. You will develop new behaviors regarding your food and your level of physical exercise that will assist you in leading a healthy lifestyle. The following behaviors may make it easier for you to keep the weight off over time.

The basic idea behind weight growth is quite straightforward: the number of calories consumed must be greater than the number of calories burned. On the other hand, as was covered in Chapter 3, both being overweight and being obese are clearly the result of a complicated set of interactions between hereditary variables, behavioral factors, and environmental factors. Despite the fact that hundreds, if not thousands, of weight-loss strategies, diets, potions, and devices have been offered to the overweight public, the multi-factorial etiology of overweight presents challenges to practitioners, researchers, and the overweight themselves in terms of identifying permanent, effective strategies for weight loss and maintenance.

There is mounting evidence that points to genetics as a contributor to the development of overweight and obesity. However, genetics cannot explain the rise in obesity that has been observed in the population of the United States over the course of the past two decades. Instead, the majority of the blame should be placed on the behavioral and environmental factors that work together to encourage people to partake in insufficient amounts of physical exercise and consume an excessive amount of food in comparison to the amount of energy that they burn. These aspects are what weight-management solutions are aiming to get a handle on and control. This chapter discusses the efficacy and safety of several weight loss strategies, as well as the combinations of weight loss strategies that appear to be connected with successful weight loss. In addition, the factors that lead to good weight maintenance will be discussed, seeing as how the challenge of keeping weight off may be a contributing factor in the prevalence of overweight and obesity. In addition, there is a brief discussion of public policy approaches that may help prevent overweight and support those who are attempting to lose weight or maintain weight loss.

CHAPTER 1

A SURPRISING FACT ABOUT FAT, HEALTH, AND DISEASE

Official dietary standards have told people for decades to eat a low-fat diet, in which fat makes up about 30% of the calories you eat each day.

Still, a lot of studies show that this way of eating is not the best way to lose weight in the long run.

Even in the biggest and longest tests, there was only a small drop in weight and no change in the risk of heart disease or cancer. But many people who support low-fat diets say that these results are wrong because the 30% fat intake advice isn't enough.

Instead, they say that no more than 10% of your daily calories should come from fat for a low-fat diet to work.

On an ultra-low-fat, or very-low-fat, diet, fat can make up no more than 10% of the calories. It also tends to be low in protein and high in carbs, with about 10% of daily calories coming from protein and 80% coming from carbs.

Ultra-low-fat diets are mostly made up of plant foods and limit the amount of eggs, meat, and full-fat dairy you eat.

High-fat plant foods, like extra virgin olive oil, nuts, and bananas, are often limited, even though most people think they are healthy.

This can be bad because your body needs fat for many important things.

It has a lot of calories, builds cell membranes and hormones, and helps your body receive fat-soluble vitamins like vitamins A, D, E, and K.

Plus, fat makes food taste good. Most of the time, a diet that is very low in fat is not as tasty as one that has a reasonable amount or a lot of fat.

Still, studies show that an ultra-low-fat diet may help with a number of major health problems in very impressive ways.

Fat is good for you in small amounts. Too much bad fat (saturated fat) in your food can make you more likely to get diseases of the heart and blood vessels.

You can do a lot of things to eat fewer bad fats. Some of them should be replaced with healthy (unsaturated) fats to keep your heart healthy and keep your weight in check.

WHAT'S THE POINT OF FAT?

For a healthy and well-balanced diet, we all need to eat a small bit of fat. The right amount of fat helps our bodies: stay warm; have energy; make hormones that help our bodies work the way they should; have essential fatty acids like Omega-3 and Omega-6, which the body can't make on its own; absorb vitamins A, D, and E, which it can't do without the help of fat.

When we eat more fat than our bodies need, the extra fat turns into body fat. We need a certain amount of body fat to work well and be physically busy. But too much fat on your body, especially around your waist, can make you more likely to get heart and blood vessel diseases. It can also make you feel more tired, hurt your joints, and cause you to snore at night.

What matters most about fat in your diet is the kind of fat you eat. In the past, people were told to eat low-fat foods, but a new study shows that healthy fats are important and good for health.

• When food companies cut down on fat, they often replace it with sugar, refined grains, or other starches. These refined carbs and starches are broken down quickly by our bodies, which can affect blood sugar and insulin levels and could lead to weight gain and illness. Instead of eating less fat, it's more important to eat "good" fats that are good for you and avoid "bad" fats that are bad for you. A good diet needs to include fat. Choose foods that are high in "good" unsaturated fats and low in "bad" saturated and trans fats.

• Monounsaturated and polyunsaturated fats, which are "good" unsaturated fats, lower the risk of getting sick. Good fats are found in foods like nuts, seeds, fish, and veggie oils like olive, canola, sunflower, soy, and corn.

• Even a small amount of "bad" fats, called trans fats, can make you more likely to get sick. Trans fats are mostly found in processed foods that are made with trans fats from oil that has been partially hydrogenated. Many of these foods no longer have trans fats, which is good news.

• Saturated fats are not as bad for your health as trans fats, but they are worse than balanced fats and should be eaten in moderation. Red meat, butter, cheese, and ice cream are all foods that have a lot of saturated fat. Some fats that come from plants, like coconut oil and palm oil, also have a lot of heavy fat.

• Instead of refined starches, eat more fish, beans, nuts, and healthy oils when you eat less red meat and butter.

ARE 'LOW FAT' AND 'LIGHTER' FOODS BETTER FOR ME?

Choosing something with less fat might not be better for you. To be labeled "lite," "light," or "lighter," a food or drink must have at least 30% less fat than the original product.

• If a food is labeled "low fat" or "reduced fat," it must have less than 3 g of fat per 100 g, and the fat amount will be shown in green on the package's label.
Sometimes, more sugar or salt is added in place of the fat to make it taste the same as the original product. This might not make the choice with less fat better for you.

Even if the food's box says it has less fat, you might want to look at the nutrition label. On the label, you can see how much "total fat" and "saturated fat" each portion has.

CHAPTER 2

TRANSFORM YOUR MINDSET TO TRANSFORM YOUR LIFE

Positive thoughts about your own health and confidence in your healthy habits may be the secret tools you need to reach your goals. A recent study found that both men and women thought they could keep up a healthy diet, but women were less sure than men that they could keep up the same level of physical activity over time, even though men reported more health problems like high blood pressure and high cholesterol.

But the study shows that no matter what gender you are, having a good view of yourself may help you get what you want. Your attitude is key. Bonnie Roney, RD, says that our thoughts and what we think to be true about ourselves have a big impact on how we act and what we do. "If we think of ourselves as active and like eating healthy foods, we're much more likely to do those things and make them habits, which is good for our health and well-being as a whole."

Get your mind in the right place to lose weight.
Many people find it very difficult to lose weight. If it were easy to lose weight, there wouldn't be so many different ways to do it. Every plan and way to lose weight has both good and bad points. But for any of them to really work, you have to have the right mindset.
Sara Riehm, a registered dietitian and certified obesity expert says, "Without the right mindset, it will be harder to start your weight loss journey and harder to reach your goals."

A family therapist in New York City named Kathryn Smerling says, "Changing your mind about how to lose weight is the most important thing you can do to lose weight." "We can't change our weight from the outside if we don't have the right inner resolve and goal."

Most people who try to lose weight do so because they want to "fix" themselves, which is the worst way to go about it. They go on diets and start working out when they don't like themselves or feel bad about themselves. All the while, they pinch their "problem" spots, call themselves "fat," and feel like they're not good enough. They focus on how to lose weight quickly and other quick fixes and lose sight of the long-term and even their own health.

"People should focus on eating a healthy, high-quality diet—as high as they can afford for themselves—and not just on the number on the scale. It is possible for the body composition to change (more muscle, less fat) without the number on the scale changing. Hunnes says, "That can be very frustrating for people." "I also think that instead of focusing on "weight loss," we should focus on health. Let's try to be our best or fittest selves, not our "thinnest" selves."

HOW TO GET IN A GOOD MOOD TO LOSE WEIGHT

• **Picture yourself losing weight**

A good place to start is to stay positive and picture yourself losing weight. You can stay motivated and on track by thinking about why you started this trip and what your life will be like when you reach your goal.

• Don't focus on your mistakes.

When you're trying to lose weight, things can go wrong, and that's totally fine. It's okay to admit that you skipped a day of light exercise or ate more calories than you planned, but try not to be too hard on yourself. Thinking badly about these mistakes can make you feel guilty, which can make you eat to feel better, which can become a cycle. Instead, tell yourself that a small mistake won't stop you from moving forward.

• Lessen the amount of stress

Having bad thoughts can be a direct result of being stressed. Try some stress-relieving activities, like going for a walk, doing yoga, taking a calm bath, meditating, or aromatherapy, to help clear your mind so you can think positively.

• Set Achievable Goals

Setting goals that are too high will make it harder to keep a good attitude about losing weight. Instead, pick small goals that are easy to reach and doable. Getting closer to these smaller goals will help you stay happy and help you see the progress you're making on your journey to lose weight.

• Celebrate your wins.

So, this brings us to the next point. It's important to celebrate every goal you reach, no matter how big or small. Not sure how to party? Read about some other ways to celebrate losing weight.

You should be your own cheerleader. Put encouraging words and quotes around your mirror to remember how far you've come. Every time you look in the mirror, you'll feel better about yourself and be more likely to think positively.

• Dress for the body you have now.

Don't ever forget how important it is to dress for your changing body. Those who have already lost some weight may feel flat and uninspired if they wear their old clothes that are too big or don't fit right. In the same way, having clothes that are too small or too tight can make you feel like a failure.

Dressing in clothes that make you feel good and strong is a quick way to keep a good attitude as you try to lose weight.

• Set up a routine that you enjoy.
It's important to get into a habit that you enjoy if you want to keep a good attitude. With an easy-to-follow diet plan, you can stay on track with your plan to lose weight. You can choose from a wide range of tasty low-calorie meal replacements, such as soups, shakes, bars, and desserts.

CHAPTER 3

FOOD CAN HELP YOU LOSE WEIGHT

To get fiber, you don't have to eat a whole bag of Grandma's prunes. The fat that goes deep in your belly can be kept away by eating leafy greens, whole grains, nuts, and beans. That's called abdominal fat, and it's the most dangerous kind because it can wrap around your liver, pancreas, and kidneys.
Visceral fat can't be burned off by "superfoods." And you can't get rid of it by doing exercises like crunches. Instead, look for ways to improve what you eat and get more exercise every day. Think about a typical week in your life. Where could you possibly make changes?

Visceral fat can be a problem for anyone, but people who need to lose a lot of weight are more likely to have too much of it. As you start to lose weight, it will help your whole body, even the fat in your belly that you can't see. You still have a chance! But limit the "saturated" fats you get from animal foods, coconut and palm oils, and full-fat dairy. Keep the serving sizes of these things smaller than you would normally. And check the labels to see how many calories and how much fat are in a dose. Look for fats that are better for you, like those from plants or fish like salmon, tuna, and mackerel that are high in omega-3s.

Sorry, but plastic surgery won't help in this case. Liposuction can't remove fat from the inside of the belly wall. So it can't get rid of the deep fat in the belly. In the same way, crash diets aren't the answer either. You're more likely to get lost. The best way to lose weight is to make changes to your life that you can keep up for a long time.

FOODS THAT FIGHT BELLY FAT

1. Avocados

Half of an avocado has 10 grams of healthy monounsaturated fats. These fats stop the spikes in blood sugar that tell your body to store fat around your middle. Healthy fats in avocado not only help keep our bellies from getting too big, but they also help our bodies better absorb carotenoids, which are found in colorful fruits and vegetables like tomatoes, carrots, spinach, and winter squash. Carotenoids are known to help fight cancer. A study from The Ohio State University at Columbus found that people who ate salads with avocado got 15 times more carotenoids.

2. Bananas

The fruit has 422 milligrams of potassium, a mineral that can help limit the amount of belly-bloating sodium in your body.

3. Greek yogurt

A cup helps good bacteria grow in your gut, which gets rid of other bugs that can cause gas.

Greek yogurt is delicious, but it is also so much more: Its combination of carbs and protein helps stabilize insulin, a hormone that tells your body to store calories as fat when levels are too high.

4. Berries

Antioxidants can improve blood flow, which gives muscles more oxygen and makes it easier to do cardio, which shows off your abs. Eat some yogurt and nuts before you go to the gym to get your muscles ready.

5. Chocolate Skim Milk

Carbohydrates and protein work together in a glass to help build muscle. Drink after a workout to get better faster. Plus, the calcium will help your bones get stronger. Not only kids drink chocolate milk.

6. Green Tea

A study in Medicine & Science in Sports & Exercise shows that drinking three cups of coffee a day may speed up your metabolism and help you burn 30 calories. The ECGC in the tea makes it easier for fat to be burned.

7. Citrus

Research from Arizona State University at Mesa says that the vitamin C in oranges and red peppers can help you burn up to 30% more fat when you work out.

8. Complete Grains

It can be tempting to think about losing weight quickly. This is especially true when new diets and social media make losing 10 pounds in 10 days seem easier than it really is. In fact, "weight cycling" or "yo-yo dieting" is linked to a higher chance of death. In reality, it's hard for many people to lose weight for many different reasons, such as their age, body type, level of physical exercise, genes, and hormones. Plus, weight is not the only thing that affects our health; it is just one of many things. Our nutrition and fitness experts would never suggest cutting calories too much or working out too much because it's bad for your health. They also say that if you do those things, you'll probably gain all the weight back faster than you lost it. The healthiest way to lose weight is, without question, to change your overall diet and way of life.

Up your veggie diet. Instead of cutting out certain foods or food groups, focus on adding a lot of healthy foods to your diet to improve your general health and help you control your weight. The water and fiber in fruits and vegetables give recipes more volume. They are also naturally low in fat and calories but high in nutrients and filling. By swapping out high-calorie ingredients for fruits and vegetables, you can make lower-calorie versions of tasty meals. You could use cauliflower rice instead of starchy white rice, or you could do a 50/50 split. If you try to make at least half of every meal vegetable-based, you'll be on the right track to better health.

- **Make a better morning meal.**

A well-balanced breakfast with fiber, protein, and healthy fats in a tasty dish will change your day, especially if you are currently skipping breakfast and still find it hard to put a healthy lifestyle first. If you don't eat breakfast, your hunger hormones may change later in the day. This could make you feel "hangry" in the afternoon, which makes it harder to avoid eating too much or giving in to urges for sugary and refined carbohydrate foods. The best, heartiest breakfasts are ones that fill you up, keep you full all morning, and keep you from getting hungry later in the day. Aim to eat between 350 and 500 calories for your morning meal, and make sure it has lean protein, full fat (like eggs, unsweetened Greek yogurt, nuts, or nut butter), and fiber (like veggies, fruit, or 100% whole grains). If you start your day with a mix of foods that keep your blood sugar stable, you will lose weight.

- **Skip sugary drinks.**

We just don't feel as full from liquid calories as we do from solid food. It's just not as enjoyable to drink juice or caramel coffee as it is to eat a bowl of stir-fry that is full of vegetables and protein. Most of the time, skipping sugary drinks is the best way to lose weight faster. As a bonus, it's also good for your heart health and can help keep you from getting diabetes. Watch how much juice, pop, sweetened coffee and tea, and alcoholic drinks you drink. If you drink each of these drinks during the day, you'll take in at least 800 extra calories and still be hungry at night. (Incidentally, alcohol may suppress the metabolism of fat, making it tougher for you to burn those calories.)

- **Get moving.**

Any kind of movement can help you lose or keep off weight. Walking is a great, cheap choice that doesn't require any other gym gear besides a good pair of shoes. A recent study found that people who took 8,200 steps a day were less likely to be overweight, have a major depressive disorder, or have other long-term health problems. So, think about walking to lose weight and improve your health in general.

Also, strength training grows lean muscle tissue, which burns more calories 24 hours a day, seven days a week, whether you're working or not. The faster you lose weight; the leaner muscle you have.

- **Eat with care.**

Slowing down and paying attention to how your food tastes, feels, looks, and smells can help you control how much you eat. But mindful eating also means paying attention to what and when you're eating. This can help you figure out if you're munching unnecessarily throughout the day, which could be adding extra calories. More importantly, try not to eat things you didn't pick out yourself. Mindful eating can help you stop letting outside authorities and cues tell you what to do and start listening to your body's own inner knowledge. Another step toward making better choices in the short and long term is to pay attention to where your extra calories come from.

- **Change things up.**

Spicy foods can help you eat less and lose weight. That's because capsaicin, a chemical found in jalapeño and cayenne peppers, may (slightly) raise your body's release of stress hormones like adrenaline, which can speed up your ability to burn calories. Also, eating hot peppers may help you eat less quickly and stop you from eating too much. You'll probably be more aware of when you're full. Ginger and turmeric are also great choices that can be used instead of hot peppers.

- **Keep track of what you eat.**

Studies show that people who keep track of everything they eat, especially while they eat, are more likely to lose weight and keep it off for the long term. A study in the journal Obesity found that the habit takes less than 15 minutes per day on average if you do it every day.

You can use an app like MyFitnessPal or a regular paper to keep track. It will keep you honest about what you've eaten. Also, when you see it written down, it's easy to see where you could use a little increase.

- **Don't let yourself skip a meal.**

Our nutritionists want to make it clear that skipping meals won't help you lose weight faster. If you're too busy during the day to sit down for a meal, keep a piece of fruit and a pack of nut butter in your car or purse, and keep snacks in your work drawer. Do whatever you can to keep from getting hungry!

Long stretches without food hurt our attempts to eat healthy in two ways: it slows down our metabolism and makes us more likely to binge later in the day. Make it your goal to eat three meals and two snacks every day, and don't go more than three to four hours without eating. If you need to, set a "snack alarm" on your phone.

- **Eat things that are full of minerals**. Potassium, magnesium, and calcium can help to counteract the effects of salt, which can cause you to get puffy. Leafy greens, most "orange" foods (oranges, sweet potatoes, carrots, melon), bananas, tomatoes, and cruciferous vegetables, especially broccoli, are all high in potassium. Low-fat cheese, nuts, and seeds can also help you feel better and get rid of gas. They have also been linked to a lot of other health benefits, like lowering blood pressure, controlling blood sugar, and lowering the risk of chronic disease in general.

CHAPTER 4

RECOVERING YOUR METABOLISM

Have you been feeling tired recently? Having urges for foods like carbs and sugar that you know aren't good for you? Having trouble getting rid of weight that won't go away no matter what you do?

Most likely, it's because of how your body works.

Your metabolism, or more accurately, your metabolic rate, is how fast your body burns calories. When your metabolism is slower than usual, it can cause a chain reaction of bad things, such as tiredness, mood swings, food cravings, and trouble losing weight.

Lucky for you, slow metabolism isn't permanent. If you make the right changes to your food and way of life, you can speed up your metabolism and start feeling better again.

And what's best? Moving in the right way doesn't take long. Follow this three-day plan to kick-start your metabolism. (and start reaping the benefits of an increased metabolic rate).

GET 8 HOURS OF GOOD SLEEP.

If you were out late on Friday night, spend Saturday morning sleeping.

When you don't get enough sleep, it can throw off the balance of hormones in your body. This slows down your metabolism and makes you more likely to gain weight. "Lack of sleep is seen by the body as an extra source of stress, so cortisol goes up and testosterone goes down," says Shawn M. Talbott, Ph.D., an exercise therapist, and nutritional biochemist.

One study from the University of Chicago found that getting only 5.5 hours of sleep each night for two weeks cut fat loss by 55%. People who sleep 6 hours a night instead of 8 hours a night usually have 5 to 15 pounds more belly fat.

Even though you can't change everything that affects your metabolism, you can change some things. Want to start over with your metabolism? Try out these ideas.

1. Eat

It might seem strange, but eating really does get your metabolism going. On the other hand, starving yourself often makes you feel worse. If you stop eating, your body slows down your metabolism to keep your weight the same. Don't forget to eat food, especially if you work out in the morning. If you eat food before you work out, it might speed up your metabolism.

2. Stick to a plan

By sticking to a routine, you can make sure you eat enough and get enough good sleep, and you can also help your natural circadian rhythm. Intermittent fasting, in which you don't eat for a set amount of time (usually 8–12 hours), may help you sleep better and keep you from gaining weight.

3. Do strength exercises.

Strength and resistance training can help you build more muscle and speed up your metabolism even when you're at rest. You don't have to lift weights either. You can also work out by using your own body weight as resistance.

4. Do some exercise

Aerobic and cardiovascular exercise can also speed up your metabolism and lower your chance of heart disease, diabetes, and other health problems. So, go for a run, try a HIIT workout, or dance all night.

5. Get moving

You can also burn calories by doing things like cleaning your house or just getting up from your work. Scientists call this NEAT, which stands for non-exercise activity-induced thermogenesis. This is your reason to take more breaks during the day at work.

6. Drink tea or coffee

Caffeine can make your metabolism go faster and has also been linked to weight loss. So drink your coffee with pride, or if coffee makes you nervous, try green tea instead.

7. Stay hydrated

Water stops you from getting dehydrated, but it may also speed up your metabolism. One study found that having a little more than six glasses of water a day may speed up your metabolism by 30% for up to 40 minutes.

8. Eat a lot of meat.

Protein builds and keeps muscle, which can help you lose weight. Because muscle is more metabolically active than fat, people with more muscle mass burn more calories on their own.

9. Add a little spice to what you eat.

Capsaicin, which is found in chili peppers, may make you feel less hungry and help you lose belly fat. They may also speed up your metabolism, which could cause you to burn up to 50 more calories every day.

10. Take it easy

When you're under a lot of stress, your body stores more fat. People who are constantly worried may notice that their metabolism slows down and they eat more. Cortisol levels can go down by getting more sleep, being more aware, or meditating.

CONCLUSION

In conclusion, weight loss is a journey that requires dedication, perseverance, and commitment. It's not just about looking good; it's also about feeling good, getting better in general, and living longer. We've looked at everything from healthy eating and regular exercise to mindfulness and meditation to lose weight in this book. We have seen that there is nobody size-fits-all way to deal with weight reduction, and that the very thing works for one individual may not work for another.

However, there are a few fundamentals that are applicable to everyone: being consistent with your efforts, making healthy choices, and remaining optimistic and motivated We have also talked about the significance of self-care, self-love, and self-compassion, as well as the requirement to be surrounded by people who are supportive and help us stay on course.

Keep in mind that losing weight is not just about losing weight; it's also about gaining self-esteem, confidence, and a fresh perspective on life. A step in the right direction is one you take toward a happier, healthier you. Therefore, never abandon yourself, remain focused, and remain committed. You deserve to live your best life and are capable of achieving your objectives.

www.ingramcontent.com/pod-product-compliance
Lightning Source LLC
Chambersburg PA
CBHW061559250726
48657CB00021B/2338